Staying Safe
with Healthy Habits

by Julie Murray

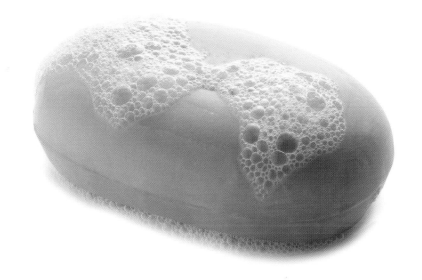

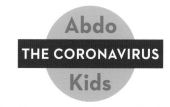

Abdo Kids Jumbo is an Imprint of Abdo Kids
abdobooks.com

abdobooks.com

Published by Abdo Kids, a division of ABDO, P.O. Box 398166, Minneapolis, Minnesota 55439.
Copyright © 2021 by Abdo Consulting Group, Inc. International copyrights reserved in all countries.
No part of this book may be reproduced in any form without written permission from the publisher.
Abdo Kids Jumbo™ is a trademark and logo of Abdo Kids.

Printed in the United States of America, North Mankato, Minnesota.

052020

092020

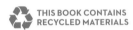 THIS BOOK CONTAINS
RECYCLED MATERIALS

Photo Credits: iStock, Science Source, Shutterstock

Production Contributors: Teddy Borth, Jennie Forsberg, Grace Hansen
Design Contributors: Dorothy Toth, Pakou Moua

Library of Congress Control Number: 2020936732
Publisher's Cataloging-in-Publication Data

Names: Murray, Julie, author.

Title: Staying safe with healthy habits / by Julie Murray

Description: Minneapolis, Minnesota : Abdo Kids, 2021 | Series: The Coronavirus | Includes online
    resources and index.

Identifiers: ISBN 9781098205546 (lib. bdg.) | ISBN 9781098205683 (ebook) | ISBN 9781098205751
    (Read-to-Me ebook)

Subjects: LCSH: Hand washing--Juvenile literature. | Social distance--Juvenile literature. | Health--Juvenile
    literature. | Hygiene--Juvenile literature. | Epidemics--Juvenile literature. | Communicable diseases--
    Prevention--Juvenile literature.

Classification: DDC 613.4--dc23

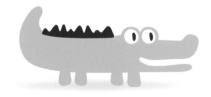

Table of Contents

COVID-19. 4

What Is a Virus?. 6

How It Spreads. 8

Healthy Habits 12

Let's Review! 22

Glossary 23

Index 24

Abdo Kids Code. 24

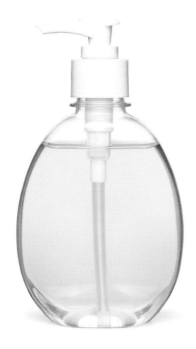

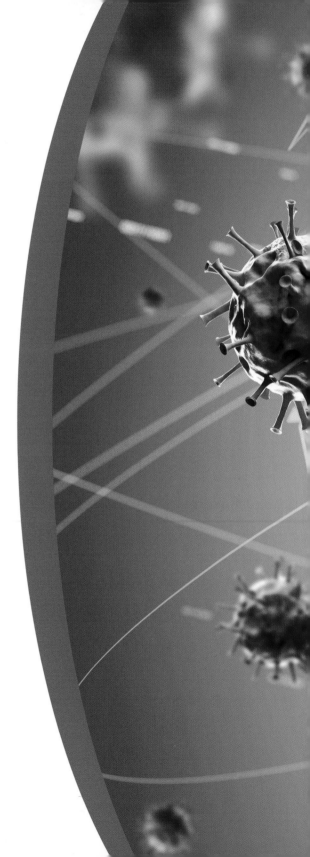

COVID-19

Coronaviruses are a large family of viruses. COVID-19 is an illness caused by a coronavirus. It spread to humans worldwide in 2020.

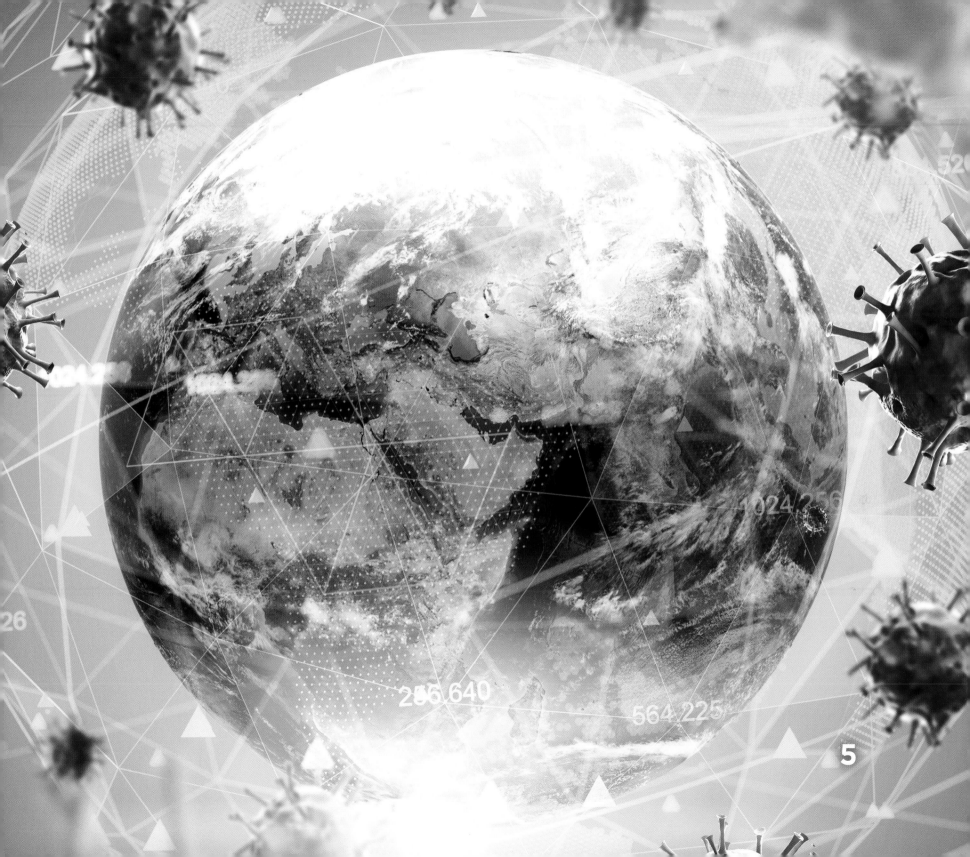

What Is a Virus?

A virus is a very tiny organism.
It needs a **host body** to survive.
If it gets into your body, it can
multiply. This can make you sick.

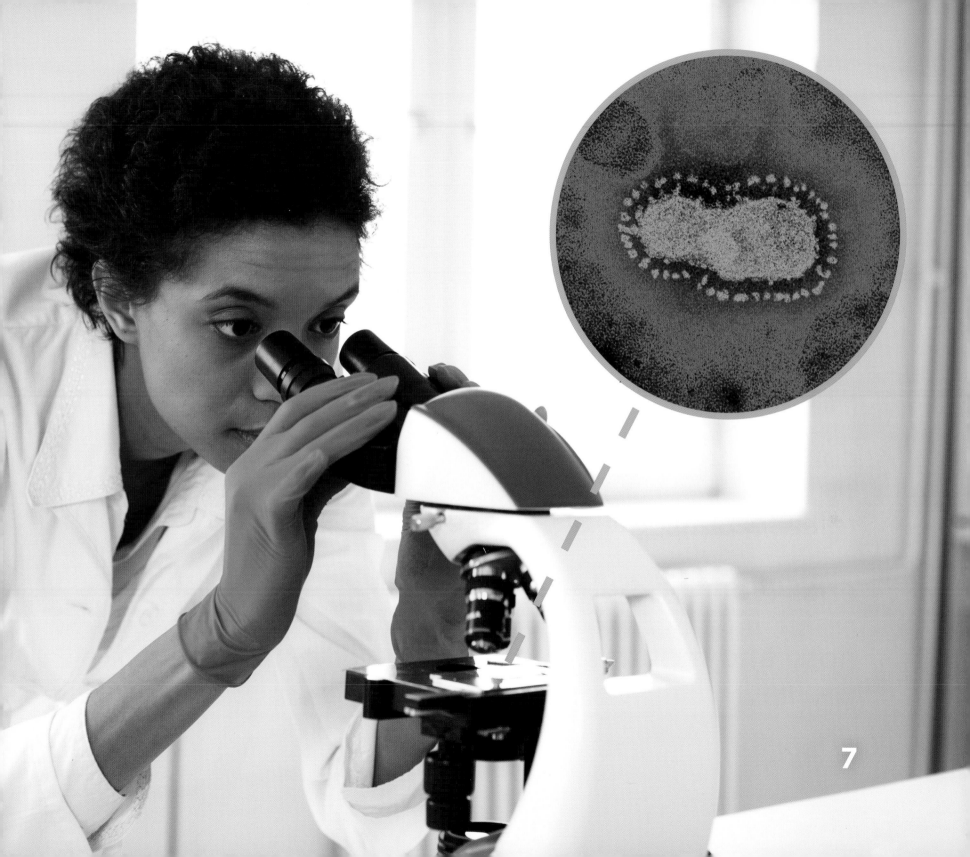

How It Spreads

A virus can spread from person to person. When someone coughs or sneezes, **droplets** are released into the air. These can enter your body through your nose and mouth.

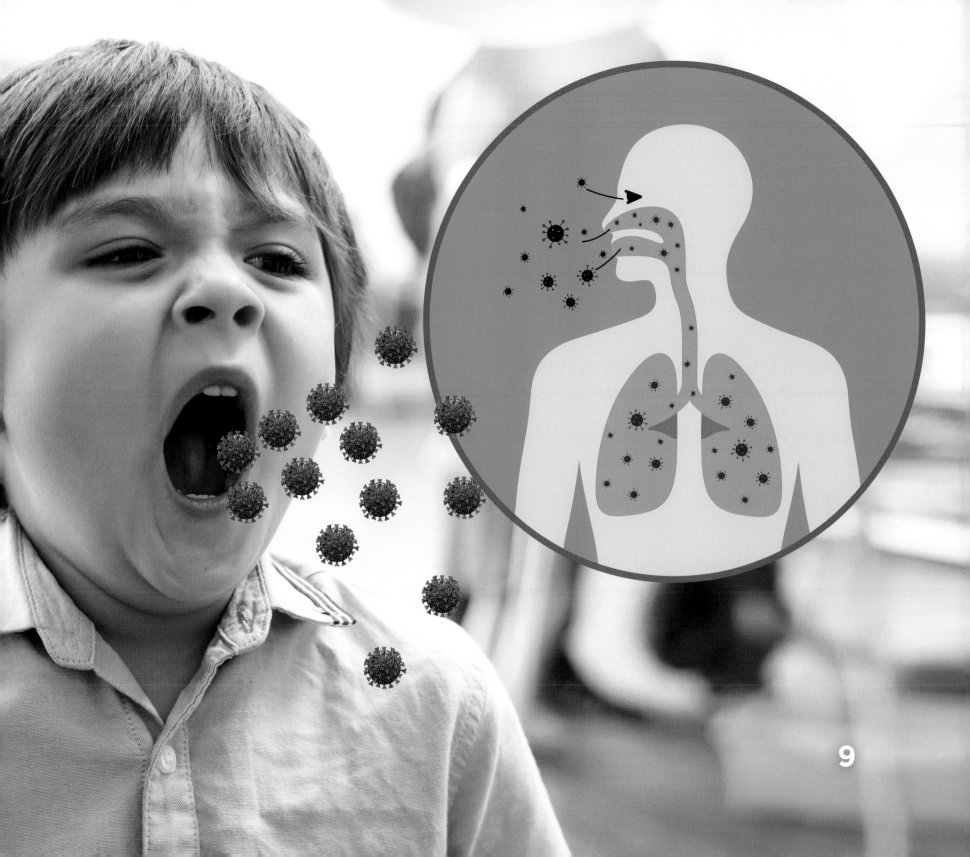

A virus can live on surfaces too. If you touch an **infected** surface, the virus can be on your hands. If you touch your face, it can get into your body.

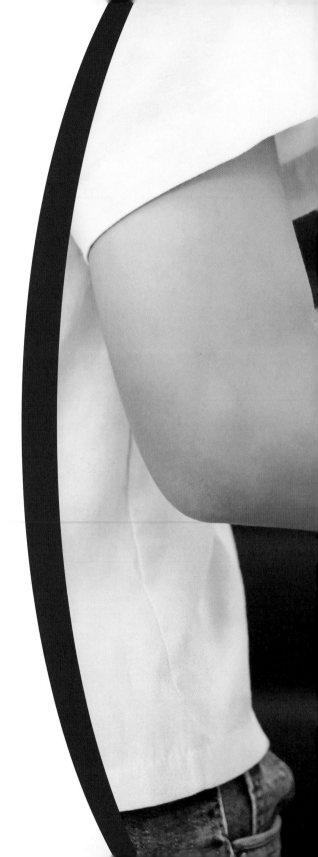

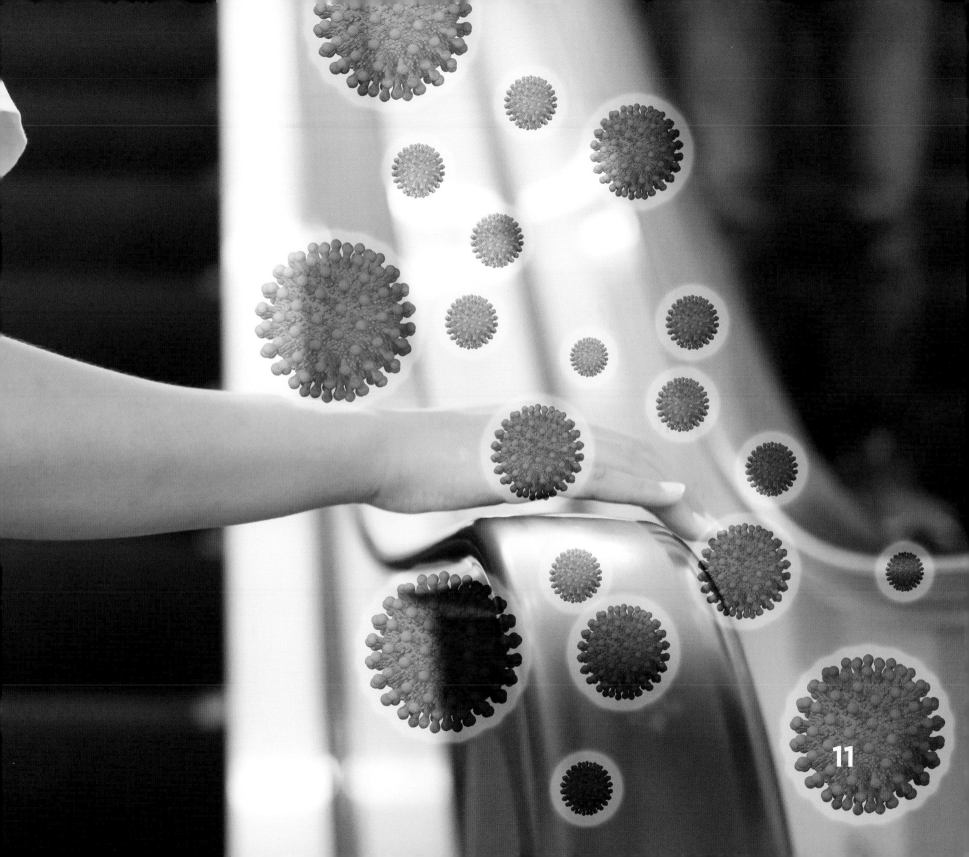

Healthy Habits

Healthy habits will keep your body strong. A strong body can help fight a virus!

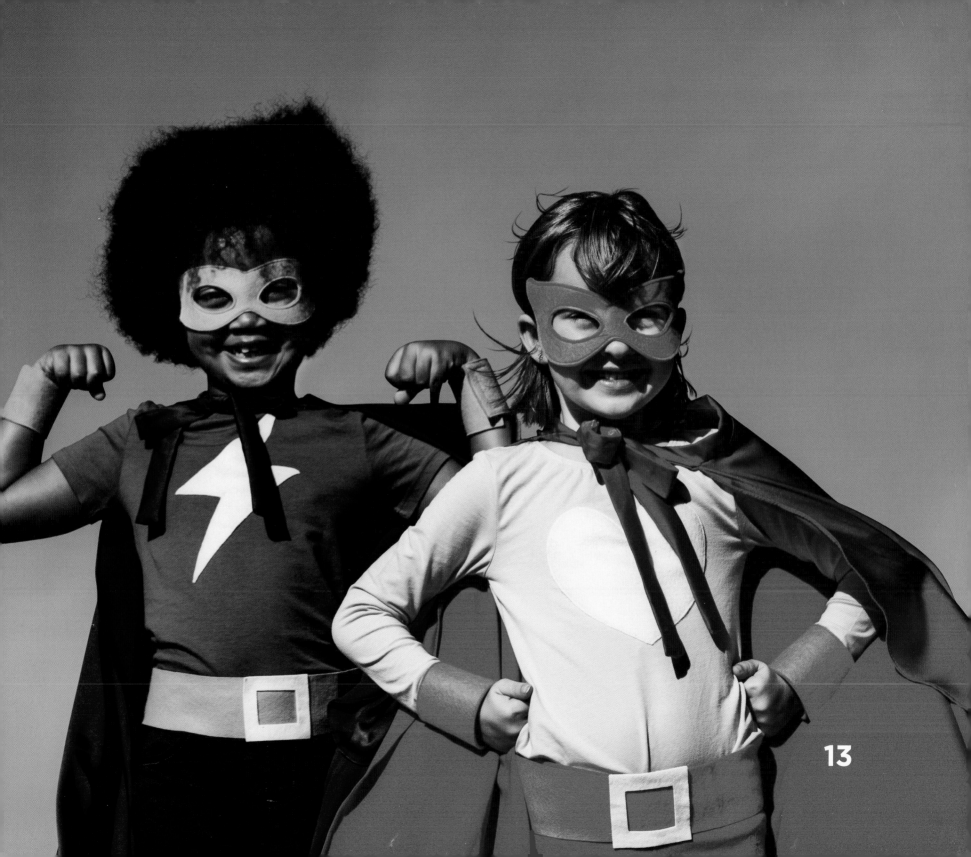

Wash your hands often! Be sure to wash for 20 seconds with soap and water. Avoid touching your face with your hands.

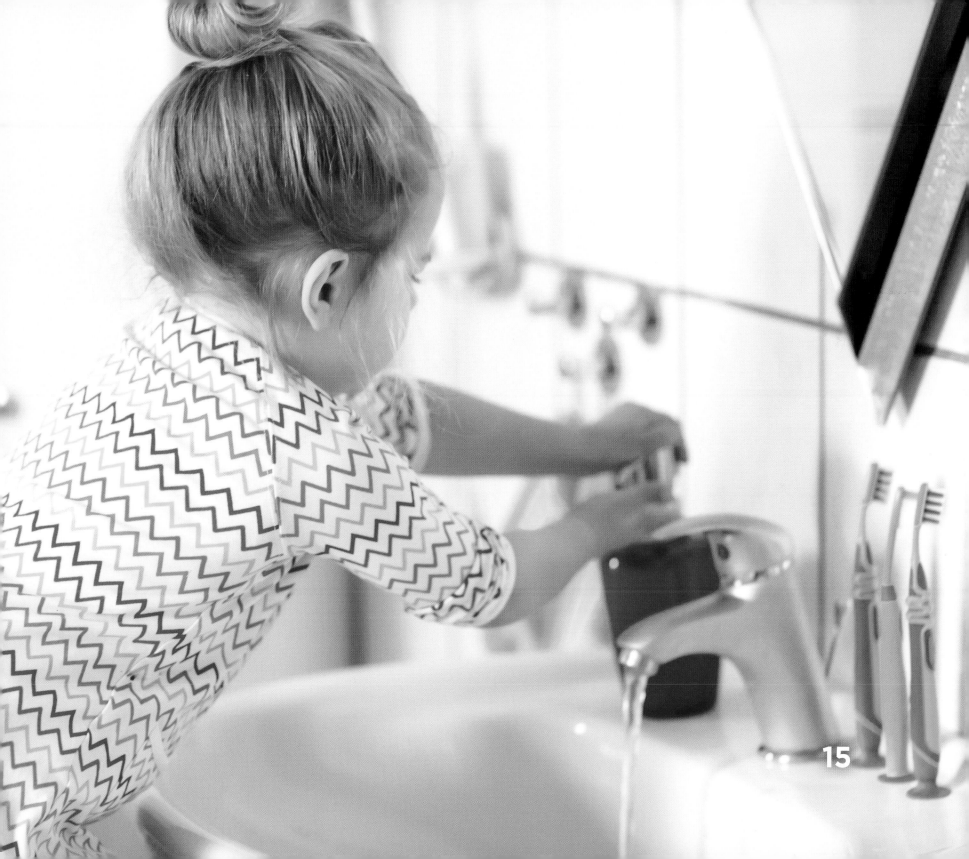

15

Eating healthy food is important.

Eat **nutrient-rich** foods like fruits, vegetables, and lean meats.

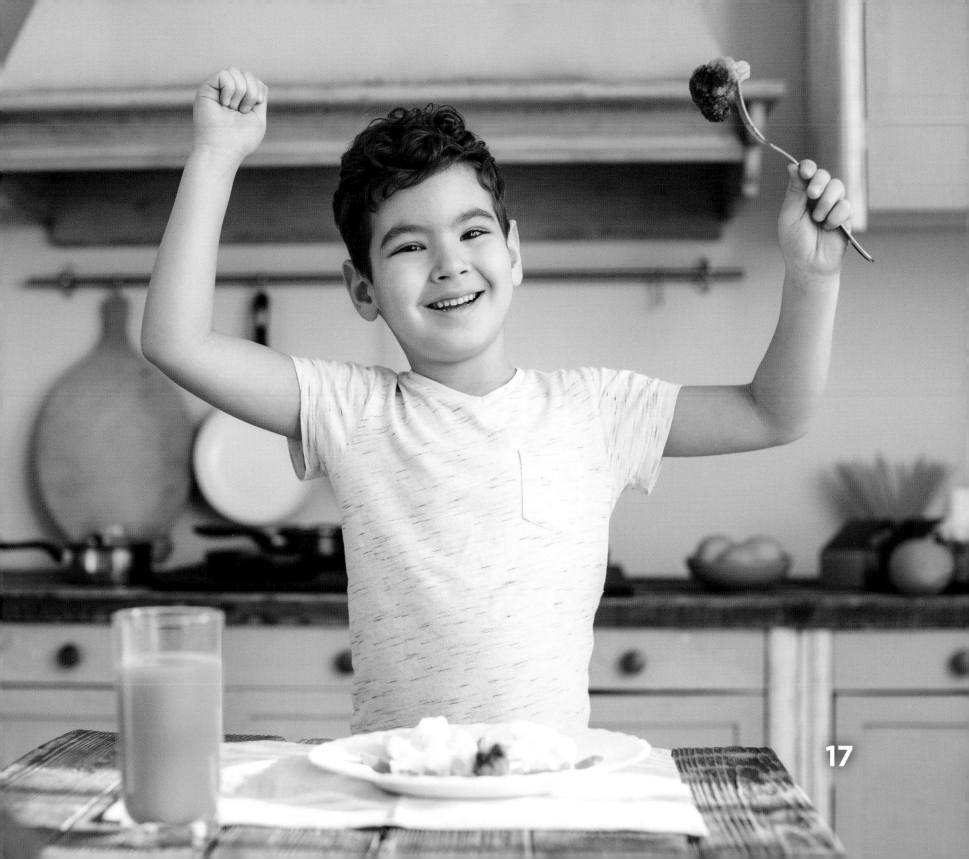

Stay active and get outside! Riding a bike or walking the dog is an easy way to get sunlight and exercise.

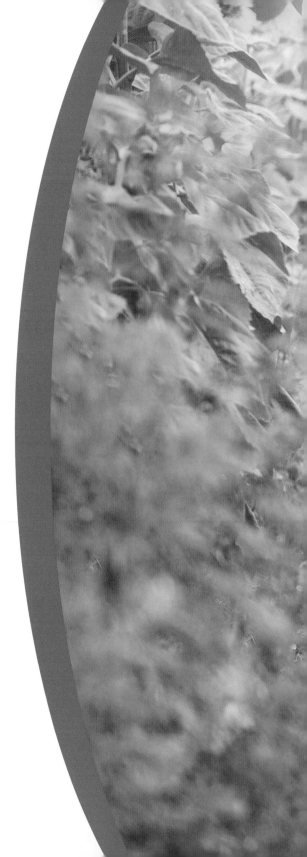

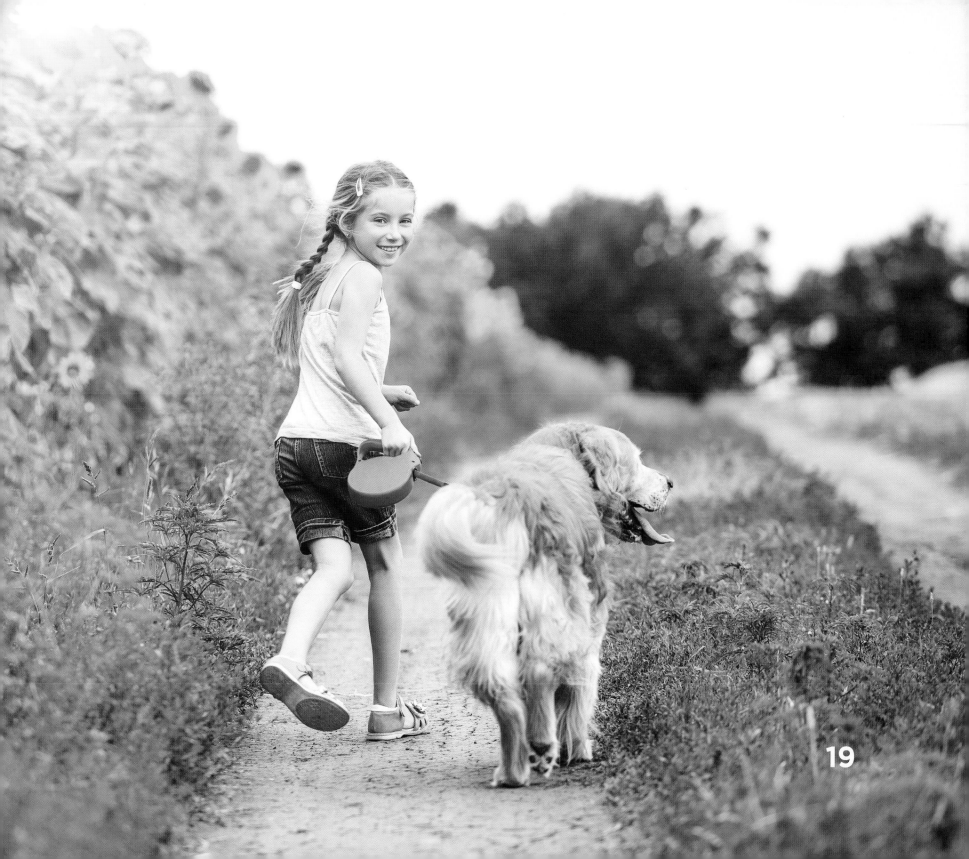

Listen to the rules that adults tell you. You might be asked to wear a mask in public. Most importantly, stay away from people who are sick. All of this helps slow the spread of a virus!

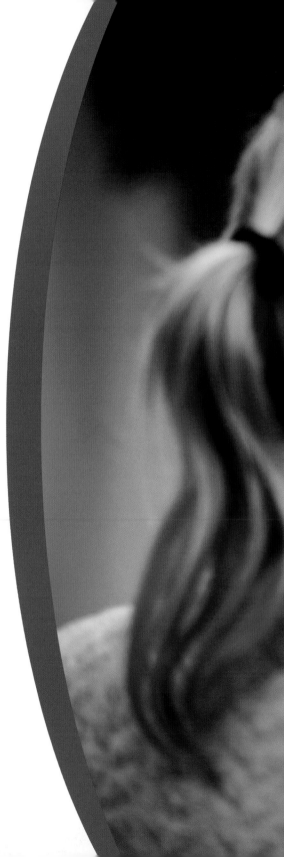

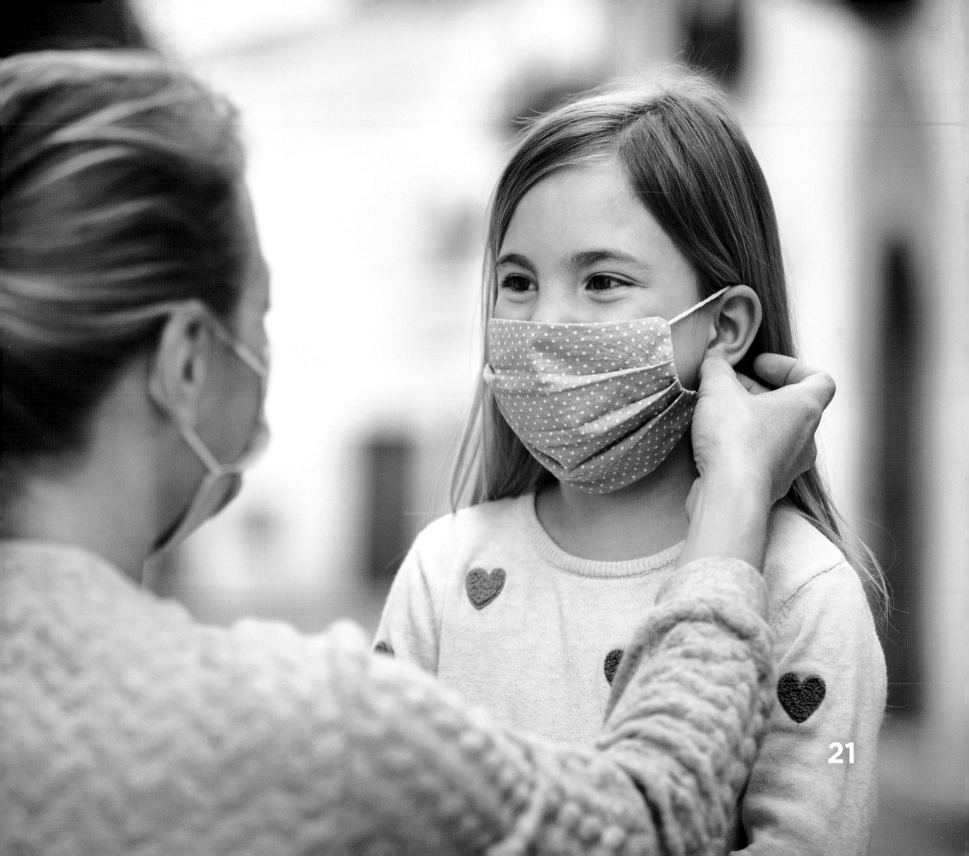

21

Let's Review!

- COVID-19 is the illness caused by a certain coronavirus. It can spread from person to person.

- If a virus gets into your body it can make you sick.

- Healthy habits keep your body strong and can help fight a virus.

- Washing your hands and staying active are healthy habits. Eating nutrient-rich foods is also a healthy habit.

- Always cover your coughs and sneezes with your arm.

- Most importantly, you should stay away from people who are sick.

Glossary

coronavirus – one in a group of viruses that cause disease. In humans, coronaviruses cause respiratory tract infections, like a common cold or a more deadly illness.

droplet – a very small drop of liquid.

host body – a living thing that is relied on by a parasite or virus for food, shelter, and other basic needs.

infected – to have caught germs or disease that was spread by someone else.

nutrient-rich – describing a food that contains a lot of vitamins and minerals, like fruits, vegetables, whole grains, and lean meats.

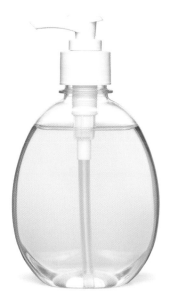

Index

coronavirus 4

COVID-19 (illness) 4

droplets 8

exercise 18

hand washing 14

healthy eating 16

prevention 12, 14, 16, 18, 20

spread 4, 8, 10, 20

sun 18

virus 4, 6, 8, 10, 12, 20

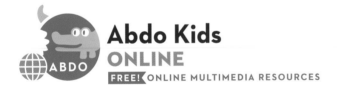

Abdo Kids ONLINE
FREE! ONLINE MULTIMEDIA RESOURCES

Visit **abdokids.com** to access crafts, games, videos, and more!

Use Abdo Kids code **TSK5546** or scan this QR code!